IMPROVING ARTHRITIS IN <u>30 DAYS</u>

Arthritis Relief within 30 Days, Recovery Plan for Long-Term Health

By Robert Redfern

About The Author

Robert Redfern – Your Personal Health Coach

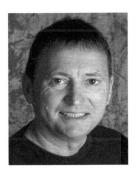

Robert Redfern (born January 1946) has helped hundreds of thousands of people in over 24 countries through online health support websites, books, radio/TV interviews, and his nutritional discoveries. His new series of books brings this work together in an easy-to-read format that everyone can follow to help resolve their chronic health problem – once and for all.

Robert's interest in health started when he and his wife Anne decided to take charge of their family's health in the late 1980s. Up until 1986, Robert had not taken much notice of his health – in spite of Anne's loving persuasion. It took the premature death of his parents, Alfred and Marjorie, who died in their sixties, to shock Robert into evaluating his priorities.

Robert and Anne looked at the whole field of health, available treatments and the causes of health problems. They found, from doctors researching the causes of disease, that lifestyle and diet were the most important contributions to health. Robert and Anne changed their lifestyle and diet and, together with the use of **HealthPoint™** acupressure, the improvement to their health was remarkable.

As well as good health, they feel and look younger and more energetic than all those years ago – before they started their plan. At the time of printing, Robert, aged 68, and Anne have every intention of continuing to be well and looking younger, using their unique understanding of Natural Health.

ROBERT REDFERN – YOUR PERSONAL HEALTH COACH
tells you everything you need to know about:

Arthritis, Osteoarthritis, and Rheumatic Diseases:

Using the Science and Knowledge of Non-Inflammatory Rehabilitation to Achieve a Pain-Free Life

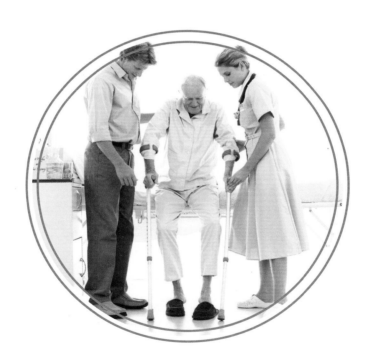

Published by

NATURALLY HEALTHY PUBLICATIONS.

From the Publisher:
This book does not intend to diagnose disease nor provide medical
advice. Its intention is solely to inform and educate the reader in
changing to and living a healthy lifestyle.

Warning:
Some information may be contrary to the opinion of your
medical adviser; however, it is not contrary to the science of good health.

CONTENTS

What Is Arthritis?   7

What Is Rheumatic Disease?   10

What Is Osteoarthritis?   11

The Western Un-Natural Food Diet   12

Can I Reverse Arthritis?   16

The Nutrients You Need   17

Why Doesn't My Doctor Tell Me I Can Get Better?   18

The Arthritis Rehabilitation Plan   19

1. Clearing Inflammation and Promoting Healing   20

2. Taking the Missing Nutrients   21

3. Immune Recovery and Strengthening   21

Optional Nutrients - but Suggested for the First 1 to 2 Months At Least   22

4. Drinking Enough Water   22

5. Avoiding Eating Unnatural Junk Foods.   22

6. Eating Real Foods   23

7. Walking and Moving Daily   27

8. Breathing Properly   29

9. Stimulating the Acupressure Points   30

10. Getting Out into the Sun As Much As Possible   30

More About Clearing Inflammation and Promoting Healing   31

More About Missing Nutrients   33

More About Immune Strengthening Formulations   34

More About Optional Nutrients   35

More About Acupressure   36

In Conclusion: 37

Sample Daily Arthritis Rehabilitation Plan   38

My Good Health Club   40

YOUR ACTION PLAN TO COMMIT TO A NON-INFLAMMATORY, PAIN-FREE LIFESTYLE

TODAY	ACTION	SIGNED	DATE
I Committed	To regaining and maintaining a non-inflammatory, pain-free lifestyle for the rest of my life		
I Committed	To drinking 8-10 glasses of water a day		
I Committed	To getting out in the sun for 20 minutes a day (except when contraindicated)		
I Read	Robert's Non-Inflammatory Arthritis Book		
I Ordered	The necessary supplements to facilitate my plan and my healing		
I Planned	My Daily Menu with **ReallyHealthyFoods.com**		
I Started	My breathing exercises		
I Started	Massaging the acupressure points		
I Reread	Robert's Non-Inflammatory Arthritis Book		
I Reviewed	The necessary supplements to facilitate my plan and my healing		
I Reviewed	My water intake		
I Reviewed	My life-giving sun exposure (except when contraindicated)		
I Reviewed	My menu		
I Reviewed	My breathing exercises		
I Reviewed	Massaging the acupressure points		
I Recommitted	To regaining and maintaining a non-inflammatory, pain-free lifestyle		
I Recommitted	To Robert's Non-Inflammatory Arthritis Book		
I Recommitted	To taking the necessary supplements to facilitate my plan and my healing		
I Recommitted	To my water intake		
I Recommitted	To following my menu		
I Recommitted	To doing my breathing exercises		
I Recommitted	To life-giving sun exposure (except when contraindicated)		
I Recommitted	To massaging the acupressure points		

What Is Arthritis?

In its strictest and purest definition, the term arthritis (derived from the Greek language) is defined as:

Inflammation of a joint or joints.

There are not just a few types of arthritis. Arthritis actually comes in many different forms, with one common factor among them all: pain. The majority of arthritis sufferers also experience inflammation as most forms of arthritis are inflammatory in nature.

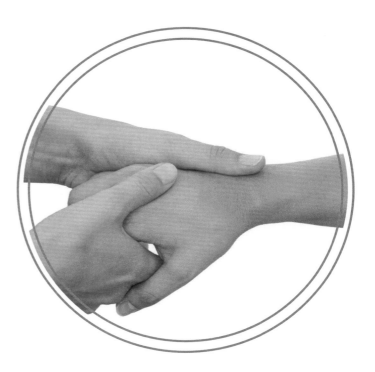

Arthritis is classified as a rheumatic disease. In addition to pain in the joints, it's often accompanied by:

- **Inflammation**
- **Swelling**

Arthritis can vary in the:

- **Region affected**
- **Pain level**
- **Damage created**
- **Length of episodes**

Who Has Arthritis?

Based on the most recent statistics:

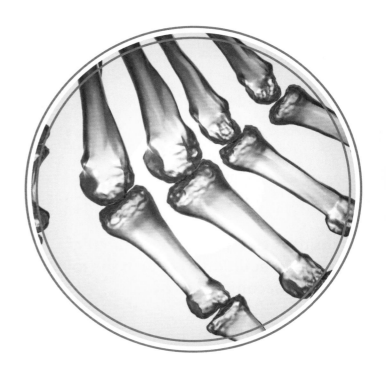

- **175 million adults worldwide suffer from arthritis.**

- **10% of the global population over age 60 has some symptoms of osteoarthritis.**

- **Osteoarthritis is ranked as the fourth leading cause of Years Lived with Disability (YLDs).**

Arthritis remains the most common cause of disability in Western countries.

20 million individuals are crippled so severely by arthritis that they have limits in daily functionality. As arthritis progresses, it inhibits physical activity and can cause many sufferers to become homebound. Numbers of arthritis diagnoses continue to increase year after year, adding up to well over 1 million hospital visits, according to Disabled World statistics.

What Does Arthritis Affect?

Arthritis affects two of the body's three types of joints.

These joints are:

1. **Synovial Joints** - Include most joints found in the body, i.e. in the limbs.

2. **Cartilaginous Joints** - Joints attached to bone by cartilage; offer very little movement.

The synovial joints are more pliable than the cartilaginous joints.

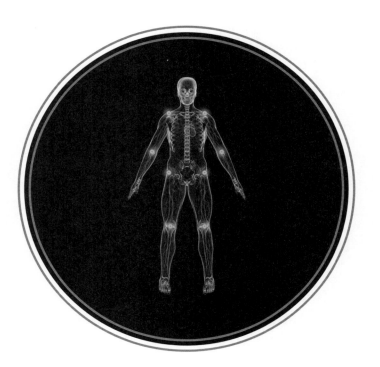

Examples of synovial joints include:

- **Shoulders**
- **Elbows**
- **Wrists**
- **Fingers**
- **Knees**
- **Hips**
- **Ankles**
- **Toes**

Examples of cartilaginous joints include:

- **Spine**
- **Ribs**
- **Pubic symphysis joint in the hips**

What Is Rheumatic Disease?

In today's society, the definition of arthritis has been expanded to include additional rheumatic disorders. These disorders not only affect the joints but the connective tissues that surround the joints and are present in other parts of the body.

Rheumatic disorders can appear out of nowhere or have a gradual onset. They are usually recognized by the pain and stiffness they create in and around single or multiple joints.

Some types of rheumatic disorders are characterized by autoimmune reactions.

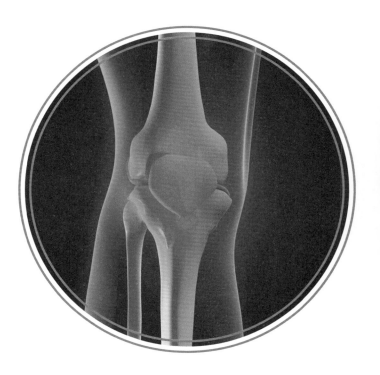

Even though there are 10 types of rheumatic diseases, those that occur most often can be put into three categories:

1. **Osteoarthritis**
2. **Inflammatory Arthritis**
3. **Extra-Articular Disorder**

We will discuss osteoarthritis in detail in the next section.

What Is Osteoarthritis?

Osteoarthritis is a degenerative joint disease. Unlike other forms of arthritis, it is non-inflammatory in nature.

Osteoarthritis affects 151 million individuals worldwide - almost 50% of those diagnosed with arthritis are diagnosed specifically with osteoarthritis.

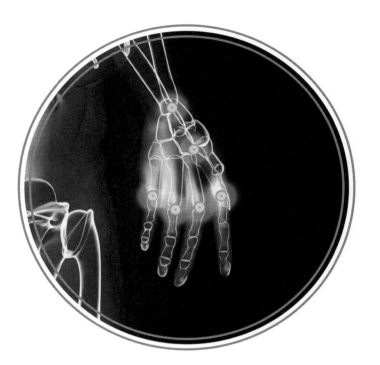

Osteoarthritis is generally thought of as a slowly progressing disease exacerbated by the aging process, accelerated by poor diet; it is extremely rare in youth. The first signs may go unnoticed as nothing more than occasional aches and pains. There are also cases where osteoarthritis does not cause pain. But in many sufferers, pain hangs around and becomes constant, sometimes even when resting.

<u>This degenerative process is due to the cartilage wearing away.</u> The body tries to repair this by rebuilding bone; however, bone spurs (bony growths that are uneven and inflexible) appear. These spurs create unnatural movements, bringing with them inflammation and pain.

There are two types of osteoarthritis:

1. **Primary:** Eating grains, cereals, and other high-sugar foods/drinks.

2. **Secondary:** Stems from an injury or other illness.

The primary joints affected by osteoarthritis are:

- **Fingers**
- **Hips**
- **Knees**
- **Neck**
- **Lower spine**

The Western Un-Natural Food Diet

In addition to non-adherence to the specific food guidelines laid out in this book, a diet that will definitely hinder one's recovery from arthritis is the <u>Western Un-Natural Food Diet.</u>

Nothing affects us more than what we choose to eat at least three to four times a day, every day.

Most of us lack the essential nutrients in our diet needed for good health, triggering inflammation. This absence of nutrients combined with one or several other unhealthy lifestyle factors can perpetuate arthritis.

The "Balanced Western Diet" (now better described as the Western Un-Natural Food Diet) is the number one disease-promoting and inflammation-producing diet in modern society. It is consumed more and more on a daily basis.

This highly inflammatory diet is made up of sugary foods in the form of breads, pastas, cereals, and potatoes. The Western Un-Natural Food Diet is far too high in unhealthy fats and lacks the antioxidants and phytochemicals that are crucial for eliminating free radicals. This all-too-common diet is lacking in high fiber foods and the foods that provide essential nutrients necessary to find relief from arthritis.

These missing foods include:

- Vegetables
- Dark skinned fruits
- Nuts
- Seeds
- Beans (except when temporarily contraindicated for recovery)

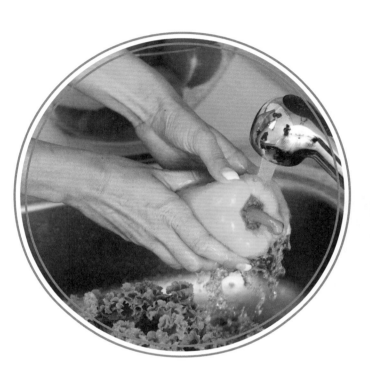

5 Eating Tips for Degenerative Disease

What you put into your body, especially when you have one or more degenerative diseases, can dictate how you feel and impact your future health.

Following some simple eating tips can support arthritis rehabilitation:

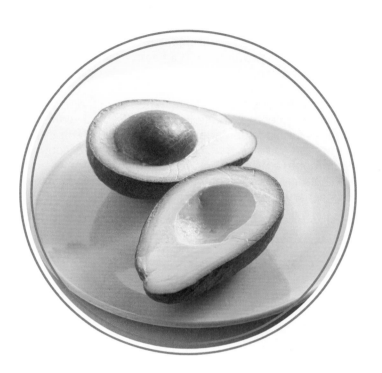

1. **Don't overeat.** Digestion requires a lot of energy the body can otherwise use for healing.

2. **Consume a high-fiber, lower-fat diet.** Saturated fats increase prostaglandin production, which creates an inflammatory state. Avoid trans-fats, hydrogenated oils, and fats in processed foods. Essential fatty acids, however, are crucial to a strong immune system, as well as to maintaining the integrity of the blood vessels. Consume monounsaturated fats in the form of moderate amounts of nuts (walnuts), seeds, and avocadoes.

3. **Simplify your diet.** Additives, hormones, and drugs run rampant in our food supply, especially in processed foods and animal products. Avoid them by eating whole foods and organic foods whenever possible.

4. **Take essential digestive enzymes.** Digestive enzymes supply enzymes for the small intestine and help with regular digestion, facilitating the breakdown of food to minimize chances of the leaky gut effect.

5. **Avoid sugar, alcohol, caffeine, and dairy.**

Broccoli Does Your Body Good

Your mother may have told you to eat your vegetables, but research now confirms that broccoli can actually benefit a serious health condition like arthritis. In a 2013 study published in *Arthritis & Rheumatism*, broccoli was proven to have potent power to fight inflammation and address the root of osteoarthritis.

When mice in the study ate a diet rich in sulforaphane (a sulfur-based compound in broccoli), they showed fewer signs of cartilage damage associated with osteoarthritis compared to mice that didn't consume sulforaphane. Sulforaphane was also proven effective to protect cow and human cartilage, potentially by blocking enzymes that trigger cartilage inflammation.

Broccoli may provide the solution to protect joints from irreversible damage caused by osteoarthritis.

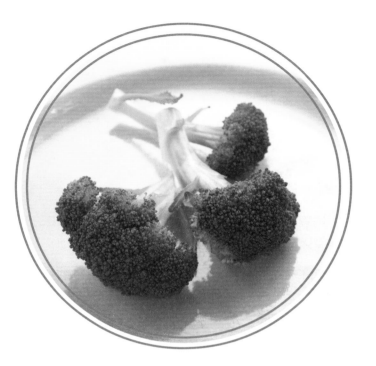

For the best results, broccoli should be enjoyed every day in a variety of ways. Blend broccoli in a daily green smoothie for extra joint protection. Liven up your salads by topping them with broccoli and other cruciferous vegetables found in sauerkraut!

Arthritis Treatment Drugs and Side Effects

Many different kinds of drugs are used in the treatment of arthritis and rheumatic diseases.

The most commonly used drugs for the relief of muscle and joint pain and the inflammation associated with arthritis are non-steroidal anti-inflammatory drugs (NSAIDs).

Common side effects include:

- **Nausea**
- **Vomiting**
- **Diarrhea**
- **Constipation**
- **Decreased appetite**
- **Rash**
- **Dizziness**
- **Headache**
- **Drowsiness**
- **Gastrointestinal bleeding**

*NSAIDs may also damage the kidneys in those with lupus.

Corticosteroids

Synthetic corticosteroids are extremely effective in decreasing the inflammation that comes with arthritis. While they do work, corticosteroids are also dangerous and compromising to overall health, suppressing the immune system even when used in small amounts.

Corticosteroids have a long list of side effects that may include diabetes, weak muscles, increased risk of infection, depression, bone loss, and much more.

Surgery may be used as a last resort to repair or replace damaged, deformed joints, relieve chronic pain, and/or alleviate the compression of nerves. With any surgery, there are risks. Infection is a primary concern, especially with arthroplasty (joint surgery). Artificial joints that are attached with pins and cement must eventually be replaced.

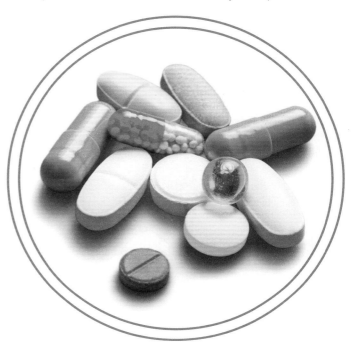

Alternatives to arthritic drugs and surgery:

- Sauna therapy/high temperature
- Massage
- Colon hydrotherapy
- Physical therapy to increase the movement of certain joints
- Stress-reducing techniques
- Hypnotherapy, EMG biofeedback, psychotherapeutic therapy
- Chiropractic care
- Relaxation techniques
- Tai Chi (controlled breathing)
- Nutritional therapy
- Rest and adequate sleep (allows the body to recuperate and increases the chances of healing)
- Acupuncture
- Hot and cold therapy

Can I Reverse Arthritis?

I do not believe it is appropriate to use the term "cure" for arthritis since most cases are brought on (or made worse) by lifestyle choices.

Cure is a medical term, and medicine does not offer any cures. (Many people argue that this is on purpose since it would put Big Pharma out of business.) However, everything has a cause. Take away the cause, apply the science of a non-inflammatory lifestyle, and your body will be able to repair itself with a little bit of help. Support tissue regeneration with a healthy lifestyle and the proper nutrients, and in the majority of cases you can become healthy again. If you call that a cure, that's up to you. I prefer to call it living a sensible, healthy lifestyle.

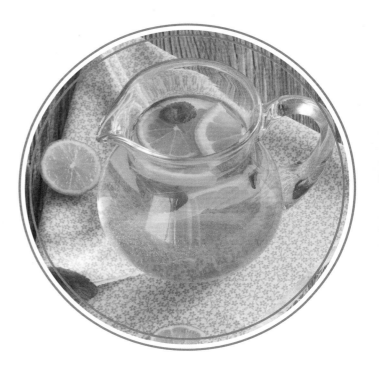

Remember, these conditions are inflammatory in nature and, therefore, will benefit from an anti-inflammatory approach. By hydrating the body {6-8 x 500ml (16oz) glasses a day} with pure, clean water and replenishing it with the proper nutrients and antioxidants in the form of vitamins, minerals, essential fatty acids, healthy carbohydrates, and amino acids, the repair and healing of the body can start to take place.

Nutritional therapy supports healing.

The initial detox can be uncomfortable but only temporarily.

Eating right can minimize the effects.

. . . regenerate with healthy lifestyle and nutrients . . .

The Nutrients You Need

Studies show that the following nutrients/therapies will help prevent or control arthritis in most people:

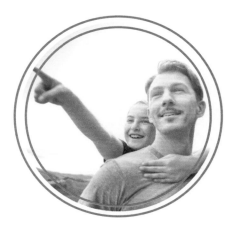

- **Microcurrent Stimulation - Electronic Acupuncture Device:** Stimulates acupressure points and gives the fastest relief in the shortest possible time; use on the points shown in the manual on **page 34.**

- **SerraEnzyme Serrapeptase, Curcuminx4000, Ecklonia Cava (Seanol), and Vitamin D3:** To support inflammation and health recovery. *(If vegetarian, see Hemp Seed Oil in the Optional section below.)*

- **Krill Oil Capsules:** Contain Krill Oil, Astaxanthin, and Omega 3, 6, and 9 Oils; simply essential for everyone.

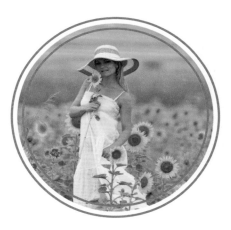

- **SAMe:** Contains SAMe Tosylate, Vitamin B6, Vitamin B12, Folic Acid, Magnesium, and a Proprietary Blend; necessary to support healthy joints and ligaments.

- **90 Vitamins/Minerals:** Full spectrum multivitamin/mineral, which you should already be taking daily.

- **Sodium Thiocyanate and Sodium Hypothiocyanite:** To clear any infection that may reside in the cells.

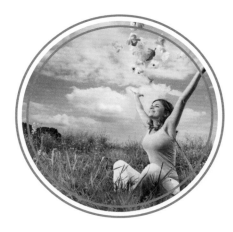

Why Doesn't My Doctor Tell Me I Can Get Better?

The Non-Inflammatory, Pain-Free Lifestyle Program can help you get better! Your doctor is obliged to conform to the drug model that is designed to maintain the monopoly that the pharmaceutical industry, the GMC in the UK and the AMA in the USA, have over all things connected with the health of individuals.

These organizations make profits by caring for sick people and do not have a business model that caters to real healthcare and recovery. They pursue a patented drug model where they can charge exorbitant prices for a lifetime of drugs that, at best, help individuals feel better and, at worse, speed up their death.

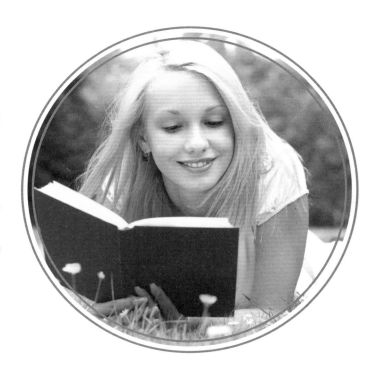

These industries are not designed to get anyone healthy, ever!

In the USA, they are shielded by the FDA and in the UK by the MHRA. The political parties and the most powerful politicians all receive money from these organizations and are responsible for making the laws that perpetuate this disease management monopoly.

When carefully followed, the Non-Inflammatory Lifestyle Program will show results within 30 days.

The Arthritis Rehabilitation Plan

Your 10 Steps to a Healthy Future

The following protocol works for any arthritic condition, to some extent.

1 Clearing inflammation and promoting healing.

2 Taking nutrients missing from food in supplement form.

3 Strengthening your immune system.

4 Drinking enough water.

5 Avoiding unnatural/junk foods.

6 Eating really healthy foods.

7 Walking and moving daily.

8 Breathing properly.

9 Stimulating acupressure points.

10 Getting out into the sun as much as possible.

It is almost unheard of for a person applying a good percentage of these lifestyle changes to their daily life to not clear their arthritis symptoms to some extent, and in many cases completely.

For details of the following suggested formulas, turn **page 31.**

1. Clearing Inflammation and Promoting Healing

Basic Plan

- **Serranol:** SerraEnzyme Serrapeptase, Curcuminx4000, Ecklonia Cava (Seanol), and Vitamin D3. Take 2 capsules x 3 times per day, 30 minutes before eating a meal with water; reduce to 1 x 3 after a good relief.

- **The Krill Miracle:** Krill Oil Capsules (better than fish oils in studies) contain Krill Oil, Astaxanthin, and Omega 3, 6, and 9 Oils. Take 1 capsule x 2 times daily. *(If vegetarian, see Hemp Seed Oil in the Optional section below.)*

2. Taking the Missing Nutrients

Advanced Plan

- **Serranol:** SerraEnzyme Serrapeptase, Curcuminx4000, Ecklonia Cava (Seanol), and Vitamin D3. Take 2 capsules x 3 times per day, 30 minutes before eating a meal with water; reduce to 1 x 3 after a good relief.

- **The Krill Miracle:** Krill Oil Capsules (better than fish oils in studies) contain Krill Oil, Astaxanthin, and Omega 3, 6, and 9 Oils. Take 1 capsule x 2 times daily. *(If vegetarian, see Hemp Seed Oil in the Optional section below.)*

- **SAM-e PLUS:** To support healthy joints and ligaments. Take 2 vegetarian Delayed Release capsules daily to aid in recovery.

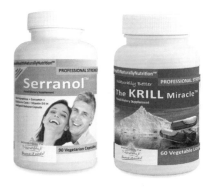

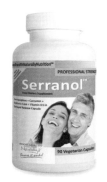
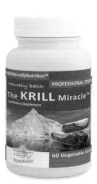
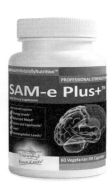

3. Immune Recovery and Strengthening

Ultimate Plan

- **Serranol:** SerraEnzyme Serrapeptase, Curcuminx4000, Ecklonia Cava (Seanol), and Vitamin D3. Take 2 capsules x 3 times per day, 30 minutes before eating a meal with water; reduce to 1 x 3 after a good relief.

- **The Krill Miracle:** Krill Oil Capsules (better than fish oils in studies) contain Krill Oil, Astaxanthin, and Omega 3, 6, and 9 Oils. Take 1 capsule x 2 times daily. *(If vegetarian, see Hemp Seed Oil in the Optional section below.)*

- **SAM-e PLUS:** To support healthy joints and ligaments. Take 2 vegetarian Delayed Release capsules daily to aid in recovery.

- **HealthPoint™:** Stimulates acupressure points and gives the fastest relief in the shortest possible time; use on the points shown in the manual on **page 34.**

- **Active Life - 90 Vitamins and Minerals:** Full spectrum multivitamin/mineral, which you should already be taking 15 ml x 2 times per day with food.

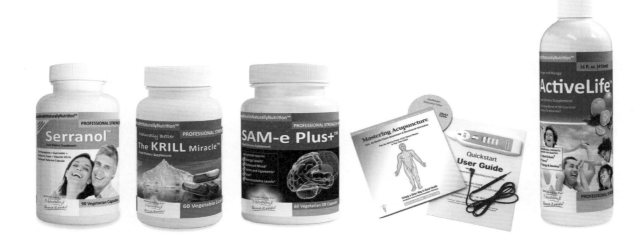

Optional Nutrients - but Suggested for the First 1 to 2 Months At Least

1st Line Immune Support: To clear any infection that may reside in the cells. In severe cases, take 1st Line at least 90 minutes after food and 90 minutes before food, approximately. Clears any infections that may reside in the cells. *Take 1 kit daily for 3 days (total of 3). 3 kits should be taken as a minimum. In serious conditions, 10 kits over 10 days are better if finances allow.*

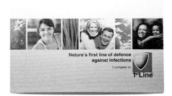

VEGETARIAN ALTERNATIVE TO KRILL OIL

Hemp Seed Oil: Contains Omega 3, 6 and 9 fatty acids from cold-pressed organic hemp. It can boost the immune system and support a positive mental state. Take 1 teaspoon x 2 times daily.

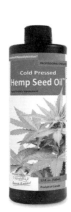

4. Drink More Water.

Drink 6-8 glasses of distilled or RO filtered water per day, with a large pinch of bicarbonate of soda (baking soda) for internal organ support.

5. Cut Out Unnatural Foods.

Until completely recovered, stop eating all starchy carbohydrates (breads, pastry, cookies, breakfast cereals, potatoes, and pasta), processed foods, and cow's milk products.

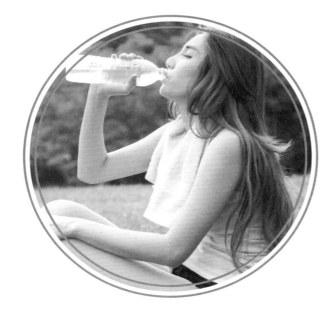

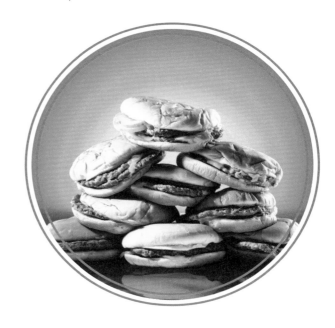

Note: Do not eat potatoes, parsnips, turnips, and rice (except for a small amount of wild or brown rice and yams/sweet potatoes).

6. Eating Real Foods

**Include some of the following foods every 2 hours for the first few months:

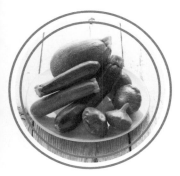

Eat 9-14 portions of fresh or frozen veggies daily (in soups, juiced, stirfried, steamed, etc.); 50% raw juiced (use the pulp in soups) and organic if possible. Blended makes for better digestion.

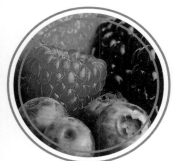

Eat 5 portions of antioxidant-rich, dark-skinned fruits (blueberries, cherries, red grapes, etc.) daily.

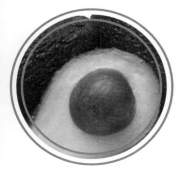

Avocados are the all-time super food with nearly a full spectrum of nutrients. If they are available where you live, make sure you have at least 2 per day for good health recovery. All arthritis issues (as well as cancer and heart disease) are helped by these.

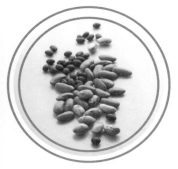

Eat 5 portions of beans, nuts, and seeds (soaked and mashed for the nuts and seeds).

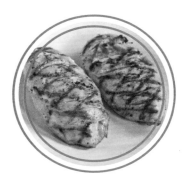

If you want to eat meat, then choose pasture-fed meats or chicken and eat only a small amount weekly. Grass-fed is healthier than grain or corn-fed animals.

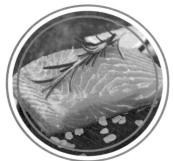

If you eat fish, then eat at least 3-4 portions per week of oily fish and vary it by choosing fish such as salmon, sardines, mackerel, etc. Even canned fish is very nutritious, and wild caught fish is best.

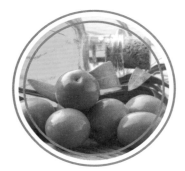

Include Hemp, Omega 3, or Krill oil and other healthy oils like Olive oil and Coconut oil.

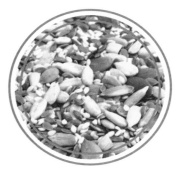

As healthy alternatives to carbs, consider Quinoa, Chia Seeds, Amaranth, Buckwheat, and Millet Seeds. Cous Cous can be used, except for those who are allergic to gluten proteins (celiacs, etc.).

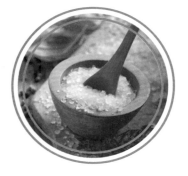

Take 3-5 (depending upon your body mass and the heat) teaspoons of Sea or Rock Salt daily in food or a little water. Sea or Rock Salt does not contain the critical mineral iodine, so add Nascent Iodine to your daily dose.

Which vegetables to eat

Note: Not all vegetables listed are available in every country.

- Artichoke
- Asian Vegetable Sprouts (Wheat, Barley, Alfalfa, etc.)
- Asparagus
- Avocado
- Beetroot
- Broad Beans
- Broccoli
- Brussel Sprouts
- Cabbage (various types)
- Capsicum
- Carrots
- Cauliflower
- Celeriac
- Choko
- Cucumber
- Dandelion Leaves
- Dried Peas
- Eggplant (Aubergine)
- Fennel
- Garden Peas
- Garlic
- Kale
- Kohlrabi
- Kumara
- Lettuce (Kos and various types)
- Mangetout Peas
- Mushrooms
- Okra
- Onions (Red and White)
- Petit Pois Peas
- Radishes
- Runner Beans
- Seaweed - all types (Kelp, Wakame, Noni, etc.)
- Silver Beet
- Spinach
- Squash
- Sugar Snap Peas
- Zucchini (Courgettes)

Which fruits to eat

Note: Not all fruits listed are available in every country.

- Apple
- Apricot
- Avocado
- Bilberries
- Blackberries
- Blackcurrants
- Blueberries
- Cherimoya
- Cherries
- Damsons
- Dates
- Durian
- Figs
- Gooseberries
- Grapefruit
- Grapes
- Kiwi fruit
- Limes
- Lychees
- Mango
- Nectarine
- Orange
- Pear
- Pineapple
- Plum/Prune (Dried Plum)
- Pomegranate
- Rambutan
- Raspberries
- Salal berry
- Satsuma
- Strawberries
- Tangerine
- Western raspberry (Blackcap)

The Garden of Eden Pyramid

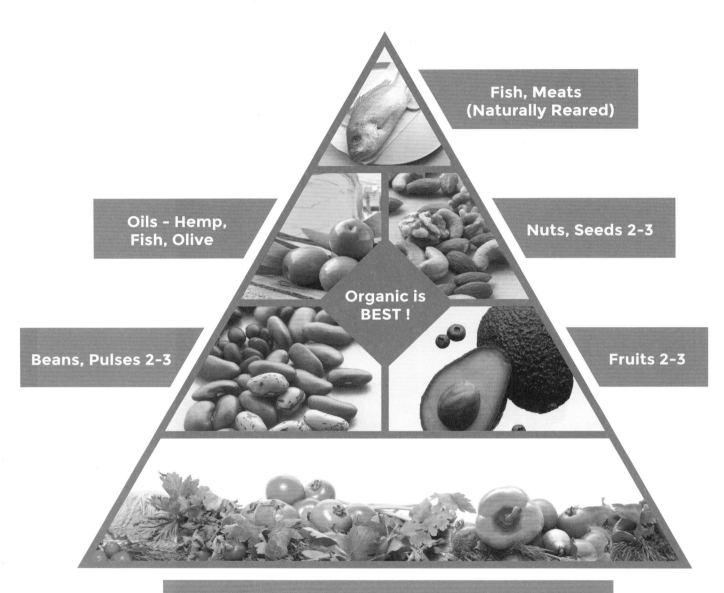

Fish, Meats (Naturally Reared)

Oils - Hemp, Fish, Olive

Nuts, Seeds 2-3

Organic is BEST !

Beans, Pulses 2-3

Fruits 2-3

Vegetables (not root): 8-12 portions per day
At least 1/2 should be raw, as in salad, etc.

7. Walking and Moving Daily

Contrary to the opinion of fitness fanatics, there are two simple ways to get your body working better and stronger. And no, they do not include swimming and cycling, although you can add these later if you want to.

One of the two simple ways to exercise is to build up to walking 3-5 miles per day, in a fast, purposely strong way with as long a stride as you can. Keep your hands moving from chest level to belt level as you move with each stride.

Use weights or wrist weights as you improve.

If this is difficult for you at the start, and your lungs are weak, then lie down to exercise to make it easier.

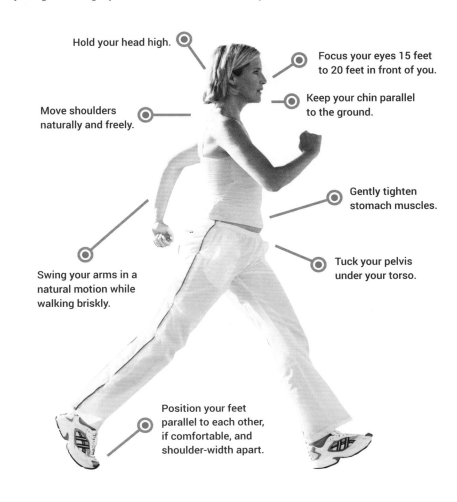

Hold your head high.

Focus your eyes 15 feet to 20 feet in front of you.

Keep your chin parallel to the ground.

Move shoulders naturally and freely.

Gently tighten stomach muscles.

Tuck your pelvis under your torso.

Swing your arms in a natural motion while walking briskly.

Position your feet parallel to each other, if comfortable, and shoulder-width apart.

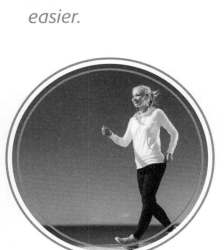

Lie down in a comfortable place. On your bed (if it's firm enough) when you first wake up is a great time and place for this. Bring a knee up to your chest as high as you can get it and then alternate with the other knee. Do as many of these as you can while keeping count. Do this every day and set yourself targets to increase the speed and the number as the weeks go by. You should be doing enough to make your lungs and heart beat faster. At the same time, as you improve your count on your back you need to be starting your walking and building this up.

The second great exercise for strengthening your lungs is to build up slowly where you can exercise at maximum rate for 2 minutes, 6 times per day. It does not matter what exercise you do, e.g. skipping, star jumps, running on the spot; just about anything, as long as your heart and lungs are working at maximum capacity. By working at maximum rate, your muscles connected with your heart and lungs will get stronger, and health will balance perfectly.

Movement is a vital part of your recovery plan.

We all know how beneficial exercise is; however, when you are in chronic pain, exercise is probably the last thing you want to do. As inflammation subsides and the body strengthens, gentle exercise can be incorporated into the treatment plan.

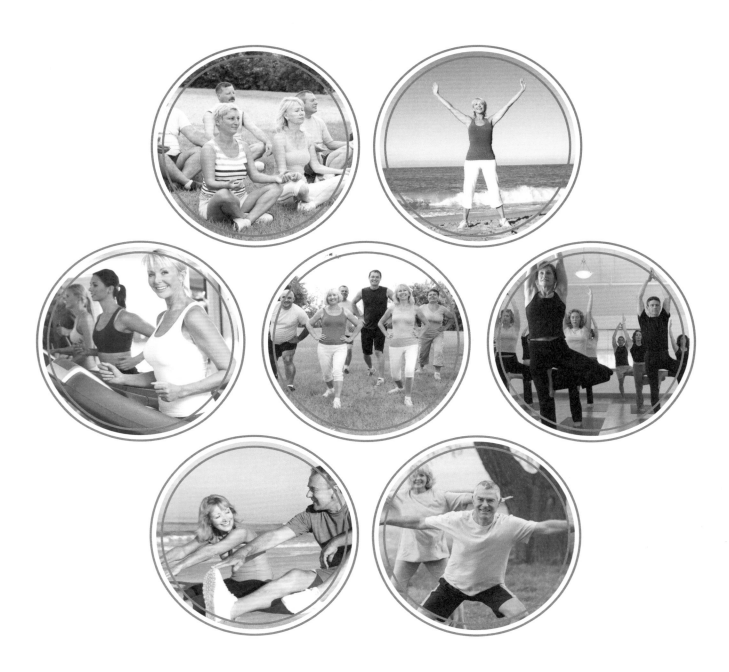

8. Learn Proper Breathing.

It is critical to breathe properly for a healthy body. Oxygen is the prime source of health.

There are two ways to breathe:

1. **Anxious Breathing: In the chest.**
2. **Relaxed Breathing: In the diaphragm or stomach area.**

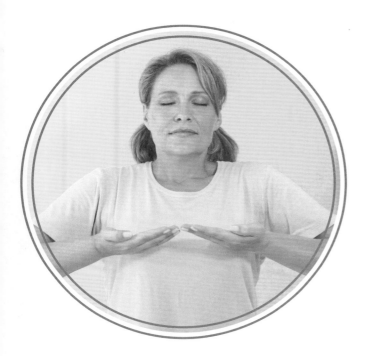

The first breath in the chest is part of the stress response and involves hormones such as cortisol. This type of breathing should last no longer than it takes to deal with a problem in life and then another hormone kicks in to create relaxed breathing. If this stress type of breathing becomes chronic or habitual, then the cortisol and retained carbon dioxide become part of the problem, and the body's natural healthy systems cannot function properly. It also weakens the immune system and opens you up to infections.

Your goal is to relearn relaxed, healthy breathing, where you clear cortisol and carbon dioxide. Too much carbon dioxide in your bloodstream destroys something called hemoglobin, which is the blood's method of carrying oxygen around the body. So it's critical to be able to breathe in a relaxed way from the diaphragm.

HOW TO BREATHE PROPERLY

The simple way to learn is to lie on your back in a firm bed or on the floor on a blanket or mat. Put a bit of weight over your belly button, such as a heavy book. Take a breath into your nose so that the book rises as you fill your diaphragm (tummy) with air. Hold the breath in your tummy for the count of 4 and then breathe out through your nose and feel your tummy deflating. Let go of any tension you may have with the out-breath. Then repeat. Your upper chest should not move at all, which shows you are relaxed and not stress breathing.

Practice over and again while lying down, and once you have really got the long, slow rhythm of relaxed breathing, then try it standing up. You may feel dizzy to begin with getting all this fresh oxygen, but you must practice this every spare minute you have.

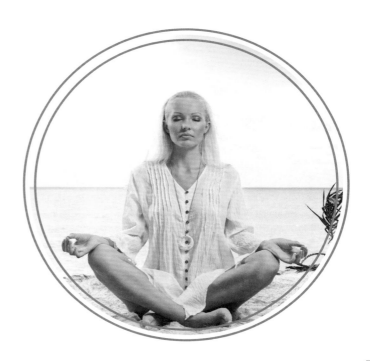

9. Stimulate Acupressure Points.

Another part of your recovery plan is to stimulate acupressure points connected to your health recovery system. There are various points that you can massage gently with your finger or stimulate with an electronic stimulator that mimics the action of acupuncture. The recommended device is **HealthPoint™**, and you can read more about this on **page 34.**

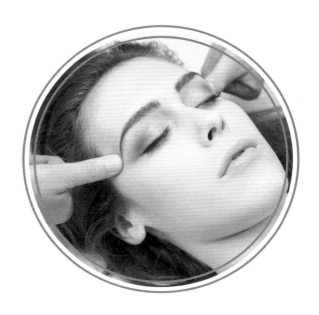

10. Getting Out into the Sun As Much As Possible

A critical vitamin for a healthy body is Vitamin D3. There is a large dose of this in the important supplement I recommend on **page 31**, but it is still important to still get some Vitamin D from the sun.

The sun is the bringer of all life, and a silly myth has developed that the sun is our enemy and we should keep out of it, or worse still, put some toxic chemicals all over us so we can go out in it.

I am not saying that we can go out on a really hot sunny day and lie in the sun for 6 hours for the first time. We are supposed to build the skin's tolerance to the sun over many weeks in the spring to stimulate protection from it, so that by the time the hot summer sun comes along we can tolerate much more.

Recommendations for sun exposure:

A: Expose as much skin as you can to the sun each day, such as on your morning walk.

B: Build up your sun exposure gradually from spring to summer seasons.

C: Try to stay out of the sun in midday without a cover-up; a cover-up is preferred to sunscreen.

D: If you do use sunscreen or sun cream, purchase organic products instead of chemical-based, name-brand creams.

E: It's important to remember that the sun is your friend and sunshine can be enjoyed in moderation!

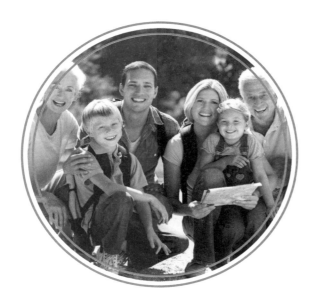

More About Clearing Inflammation and Promoting Healing

Super Nutrient Serranol™

Super Nutrient Serranol™ offers professional strength support for healthy joints, cells, heart, blood flow, circulation, and cholesterol with ingredients like:

- **Serrapeptidase** (technically Serriatia Peptidase) is a multi-functional proteolytic enzyme that dissolves non-living tissues, such as scarring, fibrin, plaque, blood clots, cysts, and inflammation in all forms − without harming living tissue. Serrapeptidase helps promote better wellbeing for your inflammatory system and supports your whole body, not only the lungs but also arteries, digestive tract, colon, joints, and anywhere blockages/ inflammation needs resolving.

- **Curcumin** (CurcuminX4000) is one of the best natural anti-inflammatory herbs to stimulate glutathione to protect cells and tissue from inflammation and help modulate the immune system. Curcumin has also been studied for its anti-bacterial, anti-viral, and anti-fungal properties.

- **Ecklonia Cava (Seanol®)** − For centuries, people throughout Asia have consumed Ecklonia Cava Extract, a species of edible brown algae. Harvested from the coastal waters off Japan, Korea, and China, all studies indicate ECE offers outstanding health benefits.

- **Vitamin D3** is critical to keep your immune system strong. The cells that make up the immune system contain vitamin D3 receptors. If there is an insufficient amount of vitamin D3 present to bind receptors, immune cells become weak and cannot protect the body from infections. Vitamin D3 deficiency is increasingly common in people of all ages because we spend less time outdoors in the sun, but this vital vitamin cannot be stored in the body. So replenishment through daily supplementation is vital to immune health.

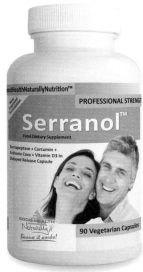

Ingredients:

- CurcuminX4000 (from Meriva®curcuma longa extract) - 250mg
- Ecklonia Cava Extract 25:1 - 50 mg
- Serrapeptase - 80,000IU
- Vitamin D3 - 1,000IU

Dosage:

Take 2 capsules x 3 times per day, 30 minutes before eating a meal with water. Reduce to 1 x 3 after a good relief.

Antarctic Pure Krill Oil

Krill are tiny shrimp-like crustaceans found in the Southern Oceans. The Southern Oceans are the only oceans in the world that remain unpolluted by the heavy toxic metals that are now found in many fish oils. Krill are a super rich source of Omega 3, 6, and 9, and their antioxidant levels are 300 times greater than Vitamins A and E and 48 times greater than Omega 3 found in standard fish oils. (Please note: People with seafood allergies should notify their physician prior to taking a Krill or fish dietary supplement.)

The unique combination of antioxidants, Omega 3, 6, and 9 oils and other potent ingredients in 100% natural Neptune-source Antarctic Pure Krill Oil offers support for:

- **A reduction in lung/heart-damaging inflammation**
- **Improved concentration, memory, and learning**
- **Improvement in cholesterol and other blood lipid levels**
- **Stabilization of blood sugar levels**
- **Healthy joints, with a decrease in pain and symptoms associated with arthritis**
- **Fighting the damaging effects of aging**
- **Protecting cell membranes**
- **Healthy liver function**
- **Bolstering the immune system**
- **Healthy mood regulation**
- **Optimal skin health**
- **Improved quality of life**

If vegetarian, see Hemp Seed Oil in the Optional section below.

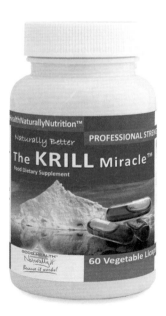

Ingredients:

- Superba™ Krill Oil - 1000mg
- Phospholipids - 450mg
- Total Omega 3 - 250mg
- EPA - 120mg
- DHA - 70mg
- Omega 6 - 15mg
- Omega 9 - 80mg
- Astaxanthin - 110µg

Dosage:

Take 1 capsule twice per day.

More About Missing Nutrients

SAM-e Plus+™

Sam-e (S-adenosyl-l-methionine) is a substance produced by our own body. It plays a central part in almost all body processes. But the older we get, the more drastically the level of SAM-e in our body decreases. Yet recent medical science has discovered and proved that SAM-e is responsible for the repair and stimulation of cell growth.

SAM-e cooperates in the repair of cells. Therefore, it is also beneficial in the case of arthrosis since it helps to repair the cartilage. This makes it an ideal product to combine with Glucosamine.

SAM-e occurs as sam-e-tosylate-disulphate (very stable). It is a completely natural product, manufactured via fermentation - now with the added benefits of magnesium, 5-htp, milk thistle extract, and chamomile flower extract. The delayed release capsules can resist the stomach acid and are only absorbed entirely in the blood when reaching the small intestine.

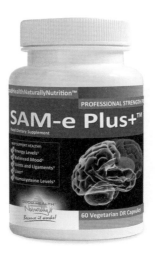

Ingredients:

- Vitamin B6 (pyridoxine HCL) - 15mg

- Folic Acid - 800mcg

- Vitamin B12 (methylcobalamin) - 200mcg

- Magnesium (as magnesium aspartate) - 15mg

- SAMe Tosylate (S-Adenosylmethionine Disulfate Tosylate) - 200mg

- Proprietary blend {Calcium aspartate, GABA (gamma aminobutyric acid), 5-htp, TMG (trimethyl glycine), milk thistle extract, chamomile flower extract} - 235mg

Dosage:

Take 2 vegetarian Delayed Release capsules daily to aid in recovery.

More About Immune Strengthening Formulations

HealthPoint

HealthPoint™ is effective on over 150 different ailments. It can be used safely by anyone – whether a young baby or senior citizen. *As with any medical device, you should always seek the advice of a qualified medical practitioner to ensure a correct diagnosis – BEFORE treating yourself.*

Stimulating the following points from the book **Mastering Acupuncture** will help to balance your health:

• **Stimulate the Cranial Electrotherapy Stimulation (CES) ear points for anxiety shown in the ear clip instructions.**

• **Stimulate the General Health Points on page 0.2.**

• **Stimulate acu-points for each painful joint shown in "Painful Disorders" points on pages 1.1-1.28.**

These points can be effectively and safely stimulated using the **HealthPoint™** electro-acupressure kit. The advantage of the kit is that it gives you the power to precisely locate the acupuncture point, and indeed other points, so you can enjoy the benefits of acupuncture at home and without any needles.

HealthPoint™ is easy to use, painless, and effective. It includes an instructional DVD and book covering over 150 pain and non-pain conditions that can be helped, such as headaches, back, neck, and joint problems.

The gentle and systematic stimulation of the body's natural healing system can speed recovery in many cases. **HealthPoint™** breakthrough technology was developed by leading pain control specialist Dr. Julian Kenyon MD 21 years ago, and today features the latest microchip technology to quickly locate acupuncture points key to specific health conditions, such as the points for arthritis.

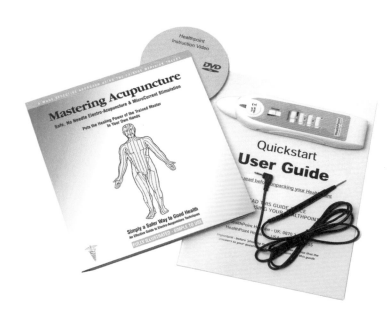

Active Life

Active Life - 90 Powerful Liquid Vitamins & Minerals is a liquid formula to ensure you get all the essential vitamins and minerals needed by your body. This single liquid supplement allows for maximum absorption and utilization of the body - 300% more absorbent than tablets!

Ingredients	Amount per Serving
Calories	39
Calcium (Tricalcium Phosphate, Citrate)	600mg
Choline Bitartrate	25mg
Chromium (Chromium Polynicotinate)	200mcg
Copper (Copper Gluconate)	2mg
Folic Acid (Vitamin B Conjugate)	500mcg
Inositol	50mg
Magnesium (Citrate Gluconate Concentrate)	300mg
Manganese (Manganese Gluconate)	10mg
Organic Seleniumethionine	200mcg
Potassium (Potassium Gluconate)	250mg
Vitamin A (Palmitate)	5000IU
Vitamin A (Beta Carotene)	5000IU
Vitamin B1 (Thiamine Mononitrate)	3mg
Vitamin B12 (Methylcobalamin)	6mcg
Vitamin B2 (Riboflavin)	3.4mg
Vitamin B3 (Niacinamide)	40mg
Vitamin B5 (Calcium Pantothenate)	20mg
Vitamin B6 (Pyridoxine Hydrochloride)	4mg
Vitamin C (Ascorbic Acid)	300mg
Vitamin D (Cholecalciferol)	400IU
Vitamin E (Alpha Tocopheryl Acetate)	60IU
Vitamin K (Phytonadione)	80mcg
Zinc (Oxide)	15mg
Ionic Trace Minerals	600mg
Phosphorus (Amino Acid Chelate)	190mg
Biotin	300mcg
Iodine (Potassium Iodine)	150mcg
Boron (Sodium Borate)	2mg
Molybdenum	75mcg
Chloride Concentrate	102mg
Amino Acid Complex	10mg
Aloe Vera Extract (200:1)	2 mg

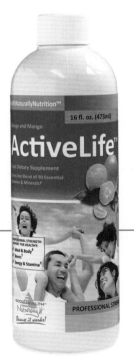

Dosage:

Take 15ml x 2 times daily with juice or water.

More About Optional Nutrients

1st Line (Thiocyanate) Immune System Support Kit

1st Line is a new all-natural product to fight against many types of infections, including viruses. It is a patented formula by a British Chemist containing Thiocyanate Ions. When added to water, 1st Line provides a drink, which forms the same molecules that make up our body's first line of defense against all types of bacteria, yeast, fungi, flu, germs, and viruses.

1st Line offers the aggressive attack to these unwanted infections without doing harm to healthy bacteria in the body, a common side-effect when using antibiotic drugs. 1st line is safe and easy to use.

Ingredients:

- Sodium Thiocyanate - 100ppm

- Sodium Hypothiocyanite - 60ppm

Dosage:

Take 1 kit daily for 3 days (total of 3). Always take at least 90 minutes before and after food.

Hemp Oil: The King of Oils

Vegetarian Alternative to Krill Miracle

Hemp is unique with an almost perfectly balanced profile of Omega 3, 6, and 9 fatty acids from cold-pressed organic hemp. Unique among common seed oil, it also contains GLA, and even more unique, it is able to raise circulating GLA. The oil may be used as part of a whole nutritional program to help maintain and improve health. With a pleasant nutty flavor, Hemp Seed Oil is ideal for use in salad dressings, mayonnaise, dips, etc. It is also ideal for massage.

Ingredients:

- Calories - 120 (500 kJ)
- Calories from Fat - 120 (500 kJ)
- Total Fat - 14.0 g
- Saturated - 1.0 g
- Trans - 0.0 g
- Polyunsaturated - 10.0 g
- Omega-6 - 8.0 g
- Omega-3 - 2.5 g
- Monosaturates - 1.5 g
- Vitamin E 1.4IU - 0.92 mg

Dosage:

Take 1 teaspoon x 2 times daily.

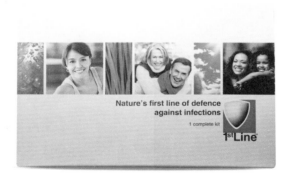

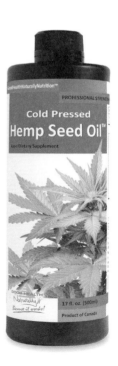

In Conclusion:

The Non-Inflammatory Lifestyle Program is a complete program, one designed to address all aspects of what is required to prevent or control your arthritis.

Arthritis is essentially a lifestyle disease, meaning if the lifestyle is changed, there is every likelihood of some recovery. With the changes in this 10 Step Plan put into effect, the body is perfectly capable of healing and recovering good health.

Drugs don't make you healthy.

Drugs do not work in that they do not make you healthy. At best, drugs will help you feel better; at worst, they will speed up degeneration and contribute to premature death.

The pharmaceutical business would prefer you continue your present, ineffective treatment plan, only utilizing toxic pills in the form of immune-suppressing drugs and avoiding the true path to prevention and healing.

You are now learning there is a better way.

The Non-Inflammatory Lifestyle Program is structured for those patients struggling to prevent or control their arthritis, even after other medical treatments have failed:

- A program that can help you learn how to love your health and improve your quality of life. The Non-Inflammatory Lifestyle Program includes treatment in the form of exercise, education, and coaching.

- A personalized program that incorporates therapy and support, assisting the person in achieving the maximum results possible.

The Non-Inflammatory Lifestyle Program is detailed within this book and, when carefully followed, will show results within weeks.

You will always end up healthier with this plan.

The worst thing that can happen with this plan is that you will get healthier but still need to take drugs if they or the disease have damaged you to the extent that you are reliant on them.

Take it all slowly and step by step.

Unless you are already used to making changes in your life, you will find adopting these habits of healthy living can be difficult to sustain. Persist. Because...

Make no mistake... Your life is worth it.

Robert Redfern, Your Health Coach

Email robert@goodhealth.nu
www.MyGoodHealthClub.com
for step by step coaching and support.

Sample Daily Arthritis Rehabilitation Plan

TIME	ACTION	AMOUNT

BREAKFAST

TIME	ACTION	AMOUNT
90 min before and 90 min after Breakfast	1st Line Immune Support	Take 1 kit daily for 3 days
30 minutes before breakfast	Serranol™	Take 2 capsules with water
Before Breakfast	HealthPoint	Stimulates acupressure points for fastest relief – use as needed
Breakfast	The Krill Miracle	Take 1 capsule
Breakfast	Active Life	Take 15ml with juice or water

LUNCH

TIME	ACTION	AMOUNT
Before Lunch	Active Life	Take 15ml with juice or water
30 min before Lunch	Serranol™	Take 2 capsules with water
With Lunch	HealthPoint	Stimulates acupressure points for fastest relief – use as needed

EVENING MEAL

TIME	ACTION	AMOUNT
Before Dinner	Serranol™	Take 2 capsules with water
Dinner	SAM-e Plus+	Take 2 vegetarian Delayed Release capsules daily
Dinner	The Krill Miracle	Take 1 capsule
After Dinner	HealthPoint	Stimulates acupressure points for fastest relief – use as needed

All the books in this series:

Fibromyalgia/Chronic Fatigue
Candida
Rheumatoid Arthritis/Juvenile Arthritis
Psoriatic Arthritis
Motor Neurone Disease
Multiple Sclerosis
Hashimoto's Thyroiditis
Human Papillomavirus
Lupus
Lichen Sclerosus
Sarcoidosis
Myasthenia Gravis
Lyme Disease
Polymyalgia Rheumatica (PMR)
Myalgic Encephalomyelitis (ME)

Other Books by Robert Redfern:

The 'Miracle Enzyme' is Serrapeptase
Turning A Blind Eye
Mastering Acupuncture
EquiHealth Equine Acupressure